Swept-Source Optical Coherence Tomography

A Color Atlas

Swept-Source Optical Coherence Tomography

A Color Atlas

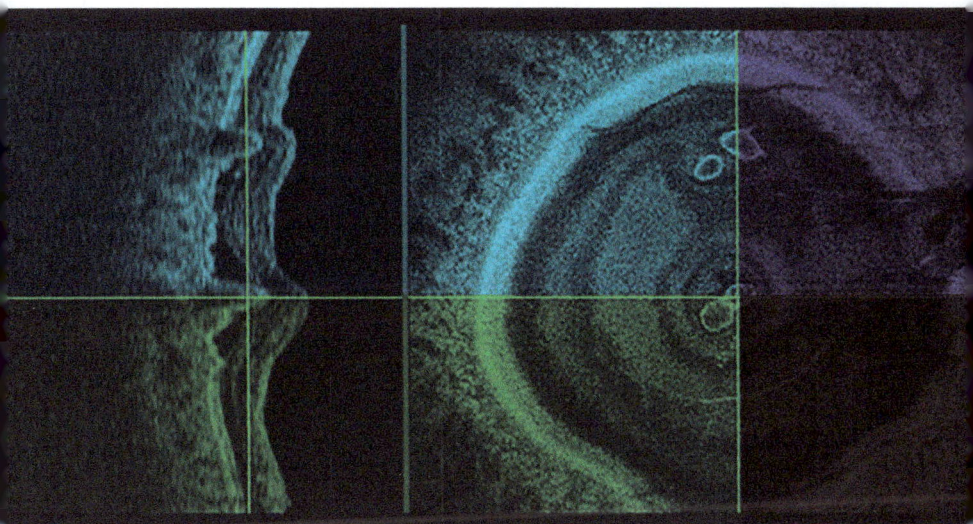

Kelvin Y.C. Teo
Wong Chee Wai
Andrew S.H. Tsai
Daniel S.W. Ting

Singapore National Eye Centre, Singapore

Edited by

Lee Shu Yen and Gemmy C.M. Cheung

Singapore National Eye Centre, Singapore

Preface by

Wong Tien Yin

Singapore National Eye Centre, Singapore

Singapore National
Eye Centre

World Scientific

Published by

World Scientific Publishing Co. Pte. Ltd.

5 Toh Tuck Link, Singapore 596224

USA office: 27 Warren Street, Suite 401-402, Hackensack, NJ 07601

UK office: 57 Shelton Street, Covent Garden, London WC2H 9HE

Library of Congress Cataloging-in-Publication Data
Teo, Kelvin Y. C., author.
    Swept-source optical coherence tomography : a color atlas / Kelvin Y.C. Teo,
Wong Chee Wai, Andrew S.H. Tsai, Daniel S.W. Ting, Singapore National Eye Centre,
Singapore ; edited by Lee Shu Yen and Gemmy C.M. Cheung, Singapore National Eye
Centre, Singapore ; preface by Wong Tien Yin, Singapore National Eye Centre,
Singapore.
       p. ; cm.
    Includes index.
    ISBN 978-9814704212 (pbk. : alk. paper) -- ISBN 9814704210 (pbk. : alk. paper)
    I. Wong, Chee Wai, author. II. Tsai, Andrew S. H., author. III. Ting, Daniel S. W.,
author. IV. Lee, Shu Yen, editor. V. Cheung, Gemmy C. M., editor. VI. Title.
    [DNLM: 1. Retinal Diseases--diagnosis--Atlases. 2. Tomography, Optical Coherence--
methods--Atlases. WW 17]
    RE551
    617.7'350757--dc23
                                                    2015020370

British Library Cataloguing-in-Publication Data
A catalogue record for this book is available from the British Library.

LIST OF CONTRIBUTORS AND EDITORS

Authors
Kelvin YC TEO
MBBS, MMed (Ophth)
Senior Resident, Singapore National Eye Centre

Chee Wai WONG
MBBS, MMed (Ophth)
Registrar, Singapore National Eye Centre

Andrew SH TSAI
MBBS, MMed (Ophth)
Senior Resident, Singapore National Eye Centre

Daniel SW TING
MBBS, MMed (Ophth)
Senior Resident, Singapore National Eye Centre

Editors
Gemmy CM CHEUNG
FRCOphth, FAMS
Senior Consultant, Vitreoretinal Service, Singapore National Eye Centre, Senior Clinician Investigator, Singapore Eye Research Institute, Associate Professor, Ophthalmology ACP, Duke-NUS GMS, Singapore

Shu Yen LEE
MBBS, MMed (Ophth), FRCS (Ed), FAMS
Senior Consultant, Vitreo Retinal Service, Adjunct Associate Professor, Duke-NUS Graduate Medical School, Adjunct Senior Clinical Investigator, SERI, Director of Undergraduate Training (Duke-NUS GMS), SingHealth Ophthalmology ACP

ACKNOWLEDGEMENTS

We are extremely grateful to the Ophthalmic imaging team at Singapore National Eye Centre for supplying the images without which this book could not have been written:

Joseph HO
Principal Ophthalmic Imaging Specialist, Singapore National Eye Centre

Paul CHUA
Senior Ophthalmic Illustration Specialist, Singapore National Eye Centre

Kasi SANDHANAM
Ophthalmic Imaging Specialist, Singapore National Eye Centre

Jackson KWOK
Ophthalmic Imaging Specialist, Singapore National Eye Centre

Vitreo-Retinal Department, Singapore National Eye Centre

Topcon Singapore Medical

PREFACE

Since the first use of film-based photography to document features of the retina in the late 1960s, ocular imaging has undergone tremendous development and advances in the last 50 years.

A major development is the optical coherence tomography (OCT), which has revolutionized our ability to visualize, measure, track and monitor subtle changes in the retina and other layers. The OCT has contributed significantly to the understanding of the normal anatomy of the eye, as well as the pathophysiology in a variety of ocular diseases. In recent years, it has become the cornerstone in the diagnosis, monitoring and treatment of the three leading causes of blindness — glaucoma, age-related macular degeneration, and diabetic retinopathy. In the latest iterations, the swept-source OCT gives us the ability to image even deeper ocular structures like the choroid and sclera with improved resolution and acquisition speed.

The SNEC Retinal Center is at the forefront of the treatment and diagnosis of vitreoretinal disorders. The SNEC Ocular Imaging Department has grown and now 25 years on, has come a long way from the overnight developing of film rolls in a makeshift darkroom to an impressive top of the line imaging suite with over 20 ocular imaging devices. The swept-source OCT represents the latest technologies we have added to our repertoire.

This book presents a compilation of images and annotations describing the microanatomical structures in both the normal and diseased eye captured on the swept-source OCT. It is written for retinal specialists and clinicians interested in retinal diseases, and is presented in a simple, atlas format to serve as a practical guide in this imaging modality. Information presented is current at the time of publishing and we hope that this book will contribute to this rapidly evolving field of ophthalmology.

Professor Tien Y Wong
MBBS, MMED (Ophth), MPH, PhD, FRCSE, FRANZCO, FAMS
Medical Director, Singapore National Eye Center

Academic Chair of Ophthalmology & Visual Sciences
Duke-NUS Graduate Medical School,
National University of Singapore

CONTENTS

1 INTRODUCTION TO SWEPT-SOURCE OPTICAL COHERENCE TOMOGRAPHY

Optical coherence tomography (OCT) is an *in vivo* non-invasive patient friendly modality for visualizing ocular structures. It produces high resolution, cross sectional images of posterior segment structures, akin to an optical biopsy.

In current ophthalmic practice, the OCT has emerged as an important ancillary test. It helps the ophthalmologist in the diagnosis of various vitreoretinal conditions and in monitoring response to treatment on follow up. The expanding role of OCT has resulted in a reduction of the number of fundal fluorescein angiography ordered.

Based on the principle of optical reflectometry, it measures the intensity and echo time delay of light that is scattered from the tissues of interest. Light from a broadband light source is broken into a reference arm and a sample arm that is reflected back from structures at various depths within the posterior pole of the eye. Backscattered light can be detected via time domain or Fourier domain methods of detection. In

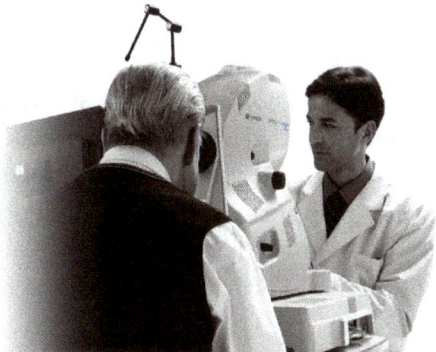

this book, we focus on the latest swept-source OCT (SS-OCT) technology, which is a form of Fourier domain detection.

In SS-OCT scanning, the light source is rapidly swept in wavelength, and the spectral interference pattern is detected on a single or small number of receivers as a function of time. The spectral interference patterns obtained as a function of time then undergo a reverse Fourier transformation to generate an A-scan image.

The features and advantages of SS-OCT include:

1. A large examination field (43°) which allows for simultaneous study of the macular area and optic nerve.
2. It utilizes a longer wavelength (1050 nm) as compared to the previous spectral domain technology (800 nm). This allows for deep range imaging which penetrates deeper to visualize the choroid and sclera in detail. It is also able to better image through media opacities, as compared to its predecessors.
3. An invisible scanning line contributes to reduced patient eye motion, enhancing successful rates of scanning and fast examination workflow.
4. A fast scanning speed 100,000 A scans per second, and faster imaging acquisition time. It takes approximately 0.01 s to obtain a B scan, and 0.9 seconds for a 3-dimensional (3D) scan.

In clinical practice, the use of SS-OCT has also allowed for better visualization of vitreous anatomy and the vitreoretinal macular interface. The inner and outer retinal layers are also more clearly defined. From a SS-OCT image, one can decipher the inner layers and the ganglion cell complex which comprises the inner plexiform layer, ganglion cell layer and nerve fiber layer. The outer retinal layers of the normal eye also shows three distinct bands. (1) retinal pigment epithelium (RPE) band which consists of the RPE, Bruch's membrane and choriocapillary network; (2) anterior to RPE band which comprises the outer limiting membrane, inner segment-outer segment line and Verhoeff's membrane; and (3) posterior to RPE band which consists of the middle and outer layers of the choroid.

Other possible examination which can be performed include:

1. Transverse or "enface" OCT. Some possible uses include visualizing the vitreo-macular interface before and after macular surgery, and to analyze different patterns of choroidal neovascular network or polypoidal choriodal vasculopathy.
2. Stereo photographs of fundus which can be obtained with the green filter.
3. Visualization of the whole retina in a 12 × 9 mm cube using the 3D SS-OCT system.

Different Modes

Analysis feature

Advanced layer detection algorithm detects 7 layers of the retina (Fig. 1.2). Thickness map and caliper function (Fig. 1.3) allow for detailed analysis.

Import function

The SS-OCT system has the ability to import color photos, fluorescein angiography, indocyanine green angiography and

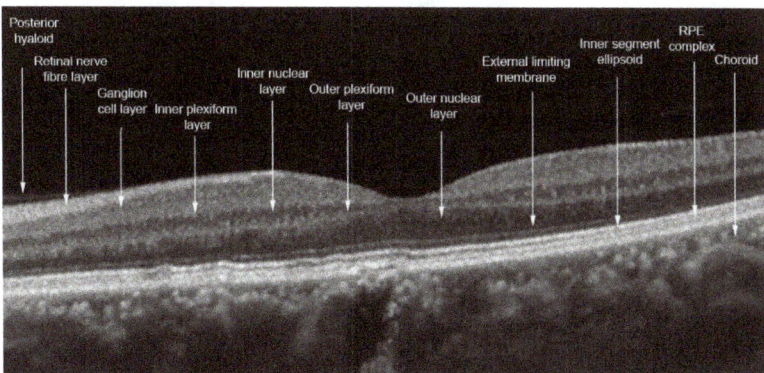

Fig. 1.1. Layers of the normal retina as seen on DRI OCT.

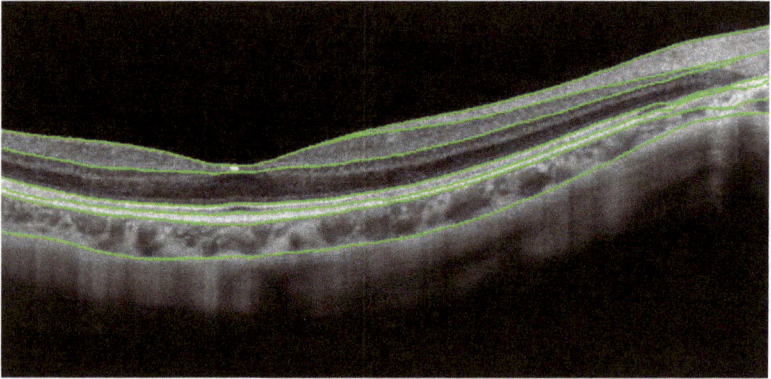

Fig. 1.2. 7-layer detection.

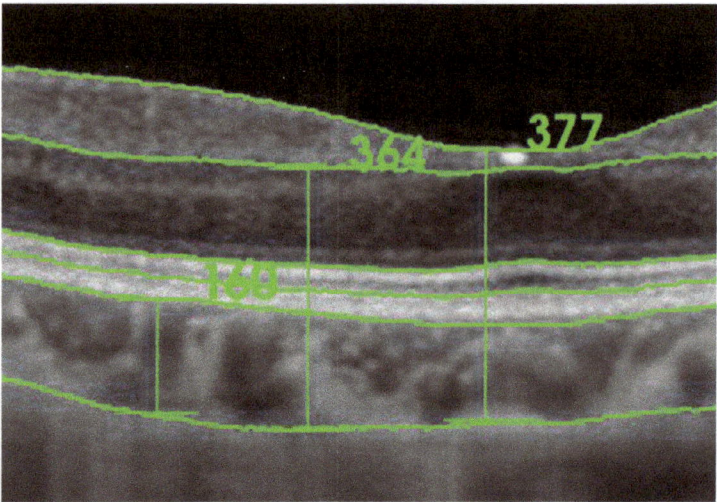

Fig. 1.3. Caliper function.

fundus autofluorescence images and compare them with OCT images (Fig. 1.4). Image overlay is made possible by recognition and alignment of retinal vessels.

3D volume rendering

Captured 3D image can be cropped (Fig. 1.5) or peeled (Fig. 1.6).

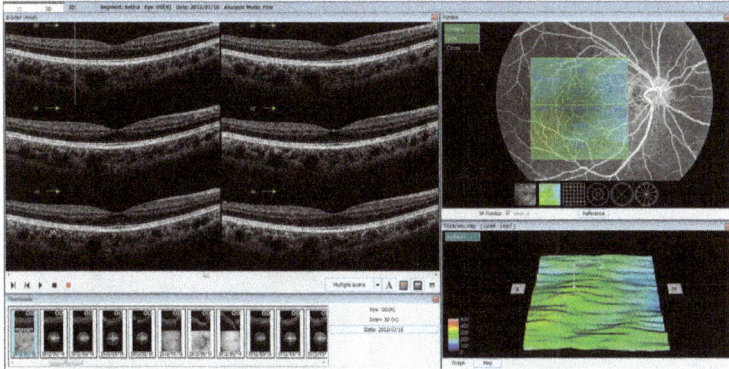

Fig. 1.4. Import function.

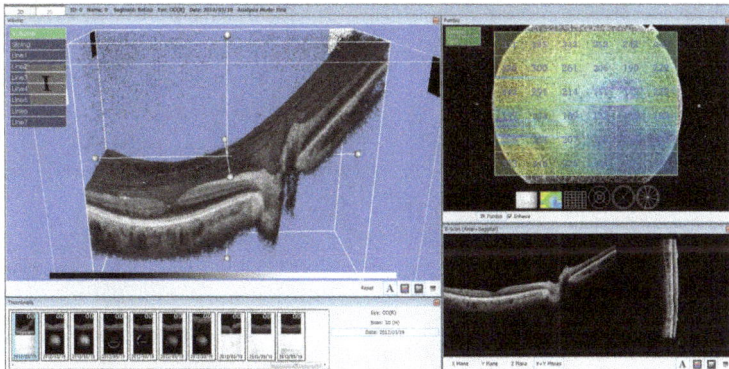

Fig. 1.5. Cropping.

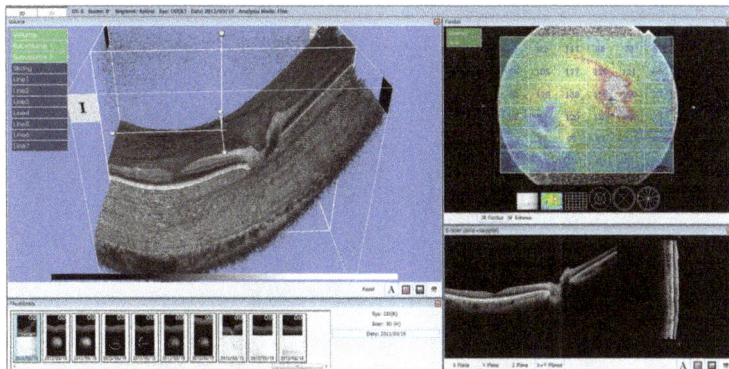

Fig. 1.6. Peeling.

Follow-up examination and comparison function

Inbuilt software detects the same scanning location of the fundus image during follow-up examination, which allows for comparison (Fig. 1.7) and monitoring of response to treatment.

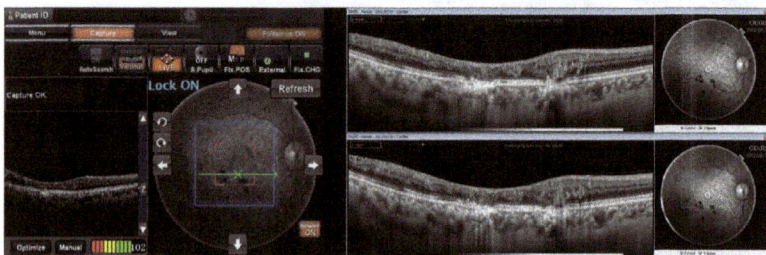

Fig. 1.7. Comparison.

2 RETINAL VASCULAR DISEASE

Diabetic Edema

Diabetic macular edema (DME) is a leading cause of visual impairment in patients with diabetic retinopathy. It is characterized by leakage of fluid and lipids from retinal capillaries, resulting in cystic retinal swelling and lipid exudation. DME was previously treated using focal laser photocoagulation, but anti-vascular endothelial growth factor

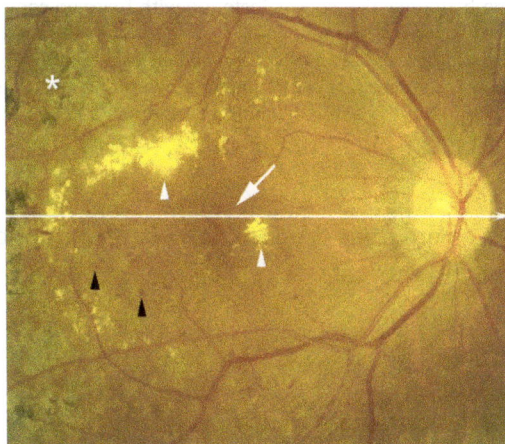

Fig. 2.1. Color photo of an eye with DME shows cystoid macular edema (*arrow*) and hard exudates (*white arrowheads*) from leaky microaneurysms (*black arrowheads*). Scars from previous laser photocoagulation can be seen (*asterisk*).

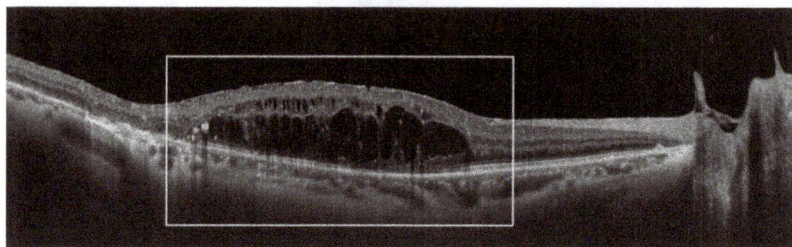

Fig. 2.2. SS-OCT (cut represented by long white arrow across Fig. 2.1) of the above patient's right eye shows multiple cystic spaces, corresponding to that seen on the color photo.

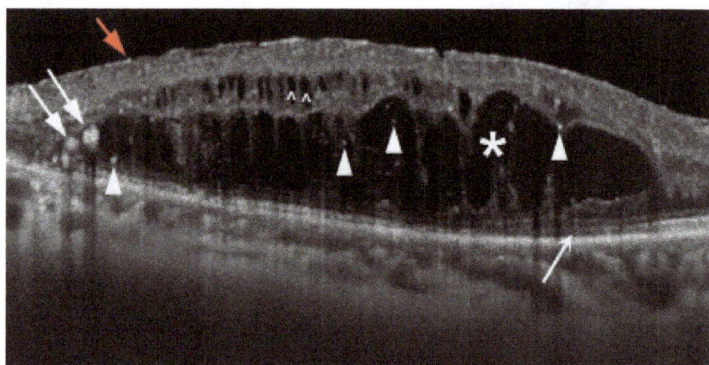

Fig. 2.3. Magnified view of the white box above. Presence of an epiretinal membrane (*red arrow*). Large hyporeflective spaces (*asterisk*) with bridging septa, mainly within the outer plexiform layer can be seen. Small cystoid spaces are seen within the inner retina (^). Hard exudates appear as hyperreflective lesions (*arrows*) with posterior shadowing. There is also the presence of multiple hyperreflective dots (*arrowheads*). Disruption in segments of the external limiting membrane and ellipsoid zone can be seen (*open headed arrow*).

treatment has emerged as the superior treatment option for visual improvement in recent years.

Retinal Vein Occlusion

Retinal vein occlusion occurs when flow obstruction occurs in either the central retinal vein or one of the branch retinal veins. It is most commonly seen as a complication of hypertensive retinopathy, where the arteriosclerotic retinal arterioles compress the retinal venules

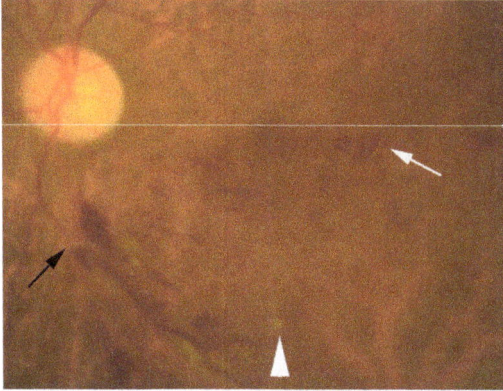

Fig. 2.4. Color photo of an eye with inferotemporal branch retinal vein occlusion. Note the presence of intraretinal hemorrhage (*white arrow*) and cotton wool spots (*white arrowhead*) in the distribution of the occluded vessel and arteriovenous nipping (*black arrow*).

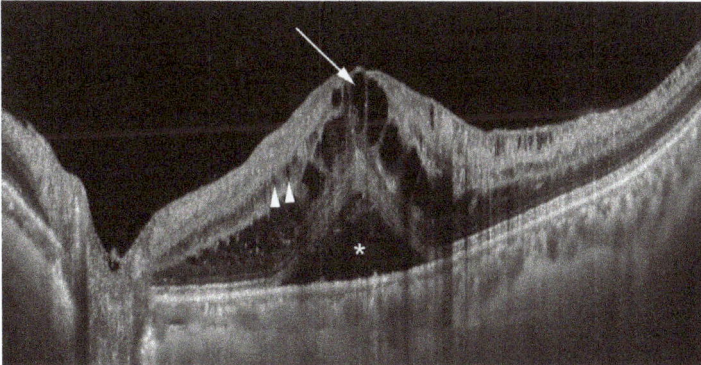

Fig. 2.5. SS-OCT (cut represented by long white arrow across Fig. 2.4) showing multiple cystic spaces separated by bridging septae from fluid accumulation predominantly in the outer plexiform layer (*arrow*). Fluid can be seen in the subretinal space (*asterisk*) and inner plexiform layer (*arrowhead*).

at an arteriovenous crossing. It is characterized by intraretinal hemorrhages and exudation in the areas of the retina drained by the obstructed vessel. Decreased vision occurs when there is macular edema or significant ischemia. Severe ischemia, if left untreated, can result in retinal neovascularization and/or neovascular glaucoma.

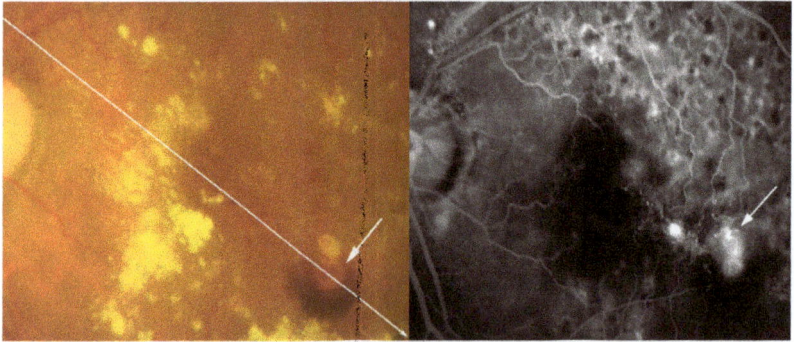

Fig. 2.6. This color fundus photo shows an eye with inferior temporal branch retinal vein occlusion which had previously received sectorial pan retinal photocoagulation. There is macular edema, hard exudates, and a localized saccular vascular malformation can be seen within the collateral vessels (*white arrow* on left image). This lesion is seen as a hyperflourescent lesion on FFA (*white arrow* on right image).

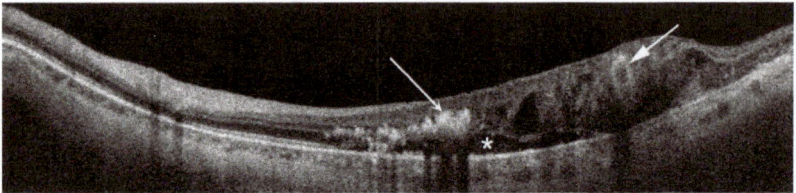

Fig. 2.7. SS-OCT (cut represented by long white arrow across Fig. 2.6) shows a round lesion with a hyperreflective wall corresponding to the vascular anomaly within the intraretinal space (*arrow*). There is macular edema (*) and hard exudates (*open headed white arrow*) resulting in acoustic shadowing.

3 MACULA DISORDERS

Idiopathic Macular Telangiectasia

Idiopathic macular telangiectasia is a group of retinal vascular disorders characterized by retinal capillary dilatation of unknown cause affecting the macula. Macular telangiectasia type 1 is characterized by aneurysmal telangiectasia associated with exudation, almost always unilateral and affecting men more commonly. Macular telangiectasia type 2 is a bilateral disease involving the macular capillary network and characterized by atrophy of the neurosensory retina. It typically

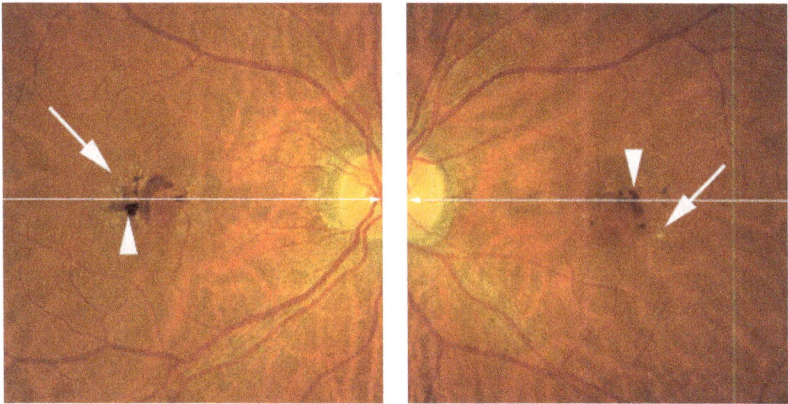

Fig. 3.1. Macular telangiectasia type 2. Note the presence of bilateral disease affecting the macular, characterized by pigment proliferation (*arrowheads*) and crystalline deposits (*arrows*).

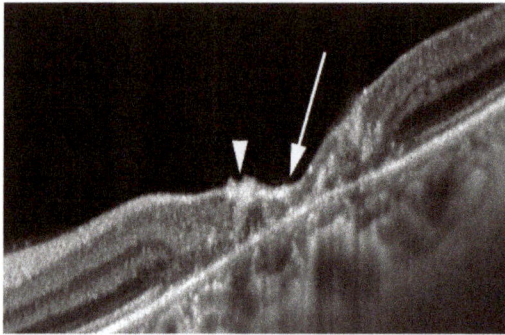

Fig. 3.2. SS-OCT scan (cut represented by long white arrow across Fig. 3.1, *left*) of the right eye shows foveal atrophy (*arrow*) with loss of the outer retina, representing a late stage of disease. Area of pigment is also seen as a hyperreflective spot (*arrowhead*).

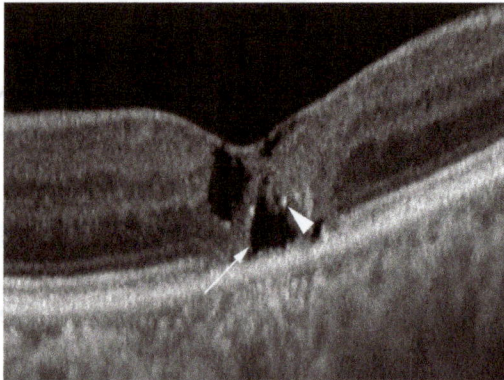

Fig. 3.3. SS-OCT scan (cut represented by long white arrow across Fig. 3.1, *right*). Note the disruption of outer retinal layers (*arrow*). The cavitations are thought to result from dysfunction or loss of muller cells. Crystalline deposits are seen as hyperreflective spots on SS-OCT (*arrowhead*).

affects individuals in the fifth or sixth decade of life with no gender predilection. It can be further classified into a nonproliferative stage where there is foveal atrophy, and a proliferative stage with the development of subretinal neovascularization.

Hydroxychloroquine Toxicity

The most significant ocular manifestation of hydroxychloroquine is bilateral pigmentary retinopathy. Early in the disease, patients can

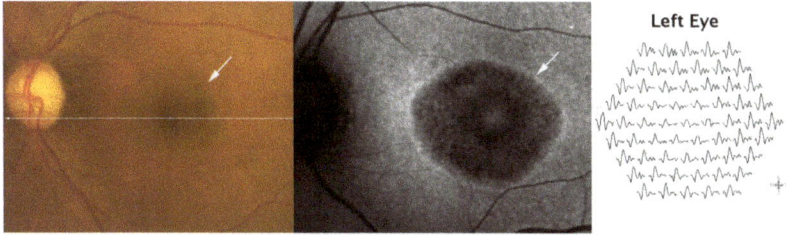

Fig. 3.4. Color fundus photo (*left*) of hydroxychloroquine toxicity showing maculopathy characterized by a parafoveal RPE depigmentation (*white arrow*). This is better appreciated on autofluorescence (*middle*) showing the true extent of the RPE damage as an increase in signal in the parafoveal region. The mfERG (*right*) responses were decreased but not delayed in the central 3 rings in both eyes. These findings demonstrate retinal dysfunction (rods>cones) with bilateral maculopathy.

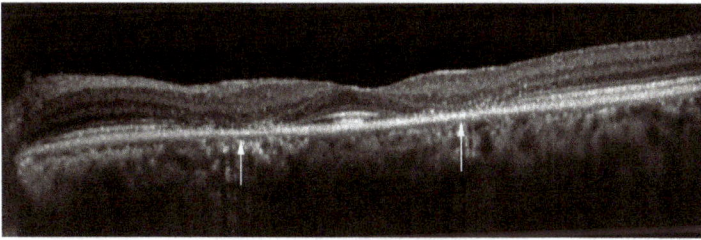

Fig. 3.5. SD OCT scan showing loss of EZ and thinning of the outer retina in the parafoveal region (*arrows*).

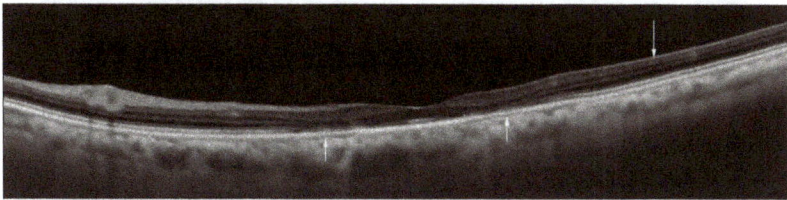

Fig. 3.6. In comparison, SS OCT image (cut represented by long white arrow across Fig. 3.4) shows the similar loss of EZ and outer retina thinning in the parafoveal region. In addition, with the longer scan, peripheral retinal atrophy can also be appreciated.

be asymptomatic with subtle paracentral scotomas. In later stages, patients can develop bull's eye maculopathy with central scotomas. End stage disease is characterized by widespread RPE and retinal atrophy with loss of central, peripheral and night vision.

Retinal Dystrophy

Macular dystrophies are characterized by bilateral visual loss and findings of symmetrical macular abnormalities. The age of onset is variable with genetic and clinical heterogeneity.

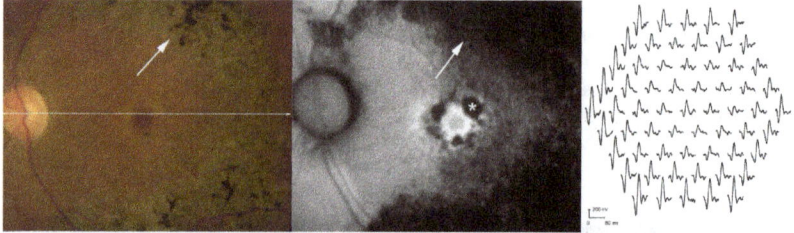

Fig. 3.7. Color fundus photo (*left*) of retinal dystrophy showing a typical bull's eye maculopathy. This is characterized by a parafoveal RPE depigmentation with sparing of the fovea center. In addition, this patient also has more peripheral retinal pigmentary changes (*white arrow*). This is better appreciated on autofluorescence (*middle*) showing the ring of decreased autofluorescence (*) bordered peripherally and centrally by increased autofluorescence. Extent of pigmentary retinopathy is better seen as areas of decreased autofluorescence (*arrow*). Responses from the mfERG (*right*) were also reduced from central 4 rings suggestive of maculopathy.

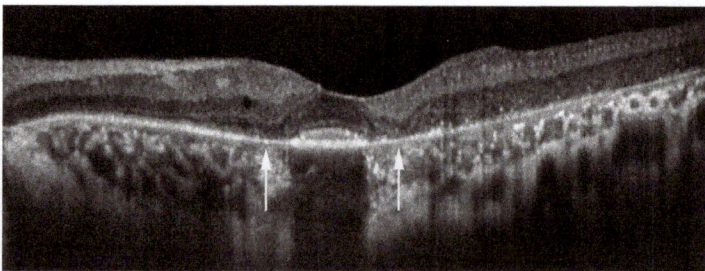

Fig. 3.8. SD OCT scan showing the parafoveal region with thinning of outer retina and loss of EZ (*arrows*). Central fovea region appears spared.

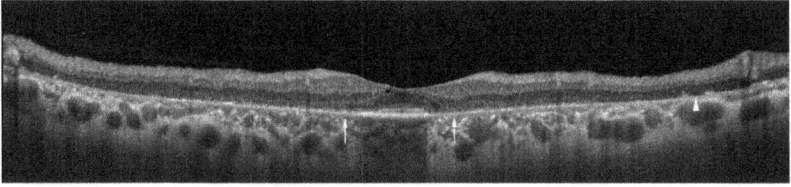

Fig. 3.9. SS OCT scan (cut represented by long white arrow across Fig. 3.7) showing a much larger extent of retina. Not only is the parafoveal region seen with similar changes noted on SD OCT (*arrows*), the peripheral retinal atrophy (*arrow head*) can also be appreciated corresponding to the areas of pigmentary change on the fundus color photo.

4 CENTRAL SEROUS CHORIORETINOPATHY

Central Serous Chorioretinopathy

Central serous chorioretinopathy (CSCR) is a disease characterized by choroidal hyperpermeability and leakage of fluid through the retinal pigment epithelium. Fluid accumulation results in neurosensory retinal detachment and/or retinal pigment epithelium detachment.

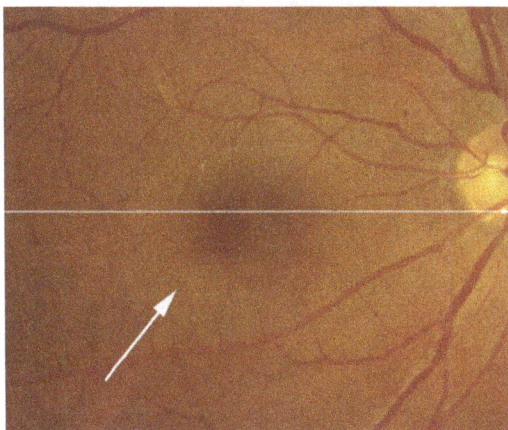

Fig. 4.1. Color photo of an eye with CSCR shows neurosensory detachment of the central macula (*white arrow*).

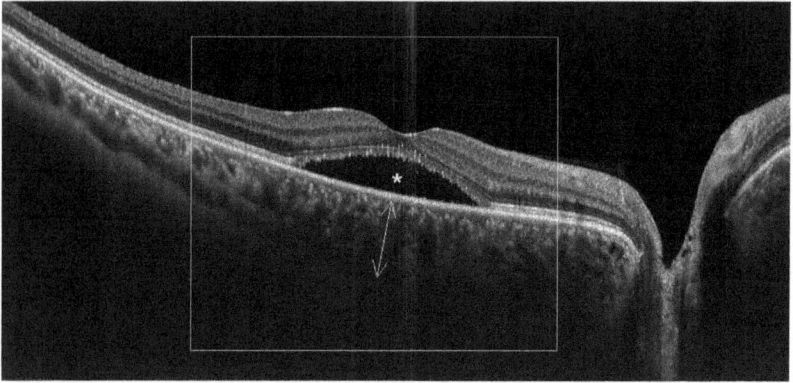

Fig. 4.2. SS-OCT scan (cut represented by long white arrow across Fig. 4.1) shows a subfoveal dome-shaped hyporeflective space between the neurosensory retina and RPE, representing subretinal fluid (*asterisk*). Note the increased choroidal thickness (*double-headed arrow*).

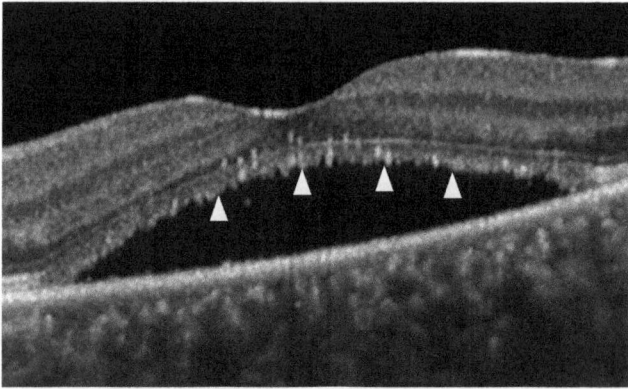

Fig. 4.3. Magnified view of box from Fig. 4.2. Small hyperreflective spots represents lipofuscin deposits, corresponding to the white spots on the color photo.

5 AGE-RELATED MACULAR DEGENERATION

Early Age-related Macular Degeneration

The dry form of age-related macular degeneration (AMD) is characterized by the presence of drusen in the macula. Drusen vary in size and characteristics. Soft indistinct drusen and pigment abnormalities are considered high-risk characteristics for development of geographic atrophy or neovascular AMD. Color fundus photograph (Fig. 5.2) shows macula of a patient with high-risk drusen with corresponding SS-OCT through the centre of the fovea (Fig. 5.1). White arrows in SS-OCT scan indicate soft drusen with overlying undulating intact RPE (Fig. 5.3).

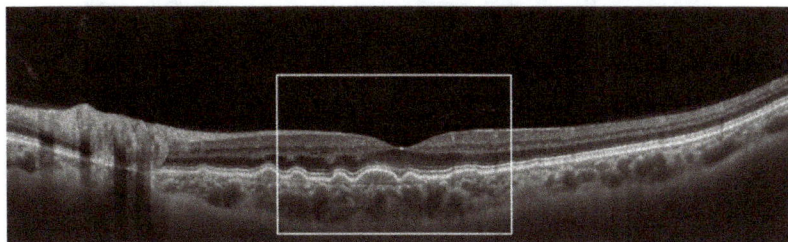

Fig. 5.1. SS-OCT scan (cut represented by long white arrow across Fig. 5.2) of a patient with drusen.

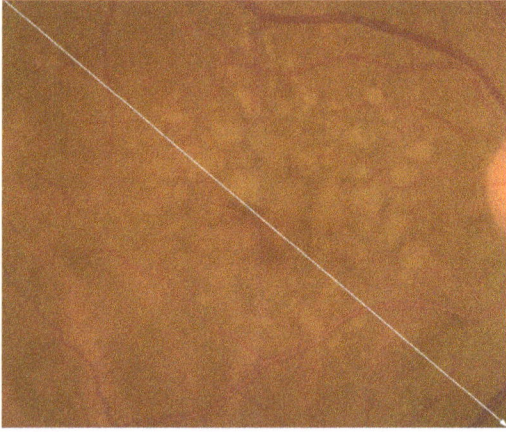

Fig. 5.2. Color fundus photo of macula with soft drusen.

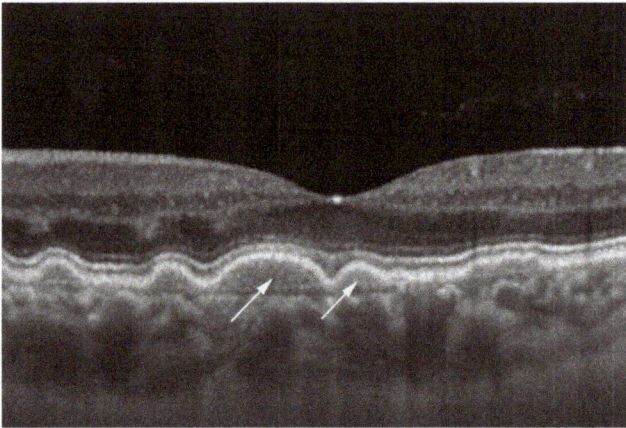

Fig. 5.3. Magnified view of white box in Fig. 5.1 showing soft drusen (*arrows*). Note the intact EZ overlying the drusen.

Late Age-related Macular Degeneration — Geographic Atrophy

Geographic atrophy (GA) is defined as a well-circumscribed area of atrophy of the retinal pigment epithelium (RPE), closure of the choriocapillaris and degeneration of the overlying photoreceptors.

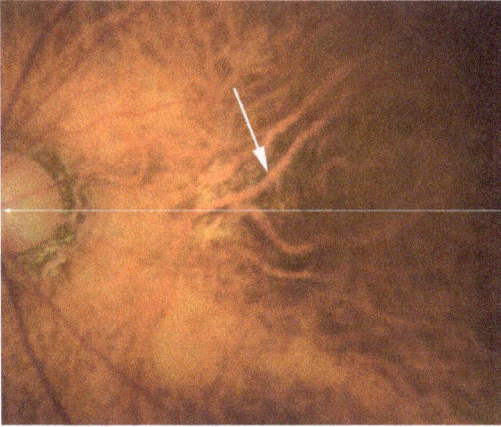

Fig. 5.4. Color fundus photo showing geographic atrophy (*arrow*). Prominent choroidal vessels can be seen as a result of RPE atrophy.

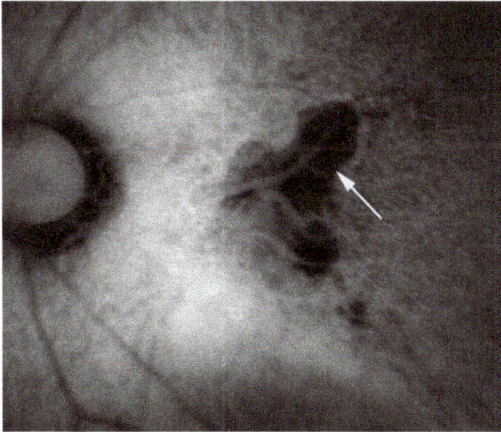

Fig. 5.5. Fundal autofluorescence reveals a hypofluorescent area (*arrow*) corresponding to the area of geographic atrophy.

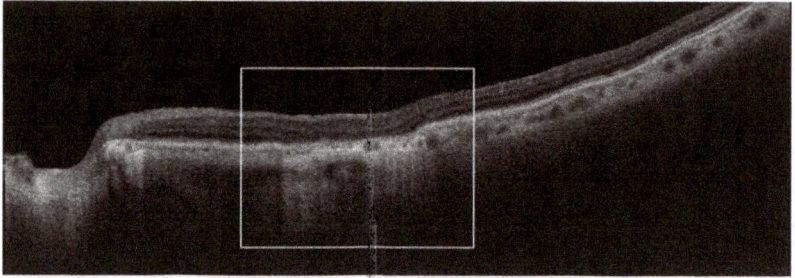

Fig. 5.6. SS-OCT scan (cut represented by long white arrow across Fig. 5.4) of a patient with geographic atrophy as characterized by loss of RPE. Within the corresponding area, increased signal from the choroid can be seen due to increased penetration of light. The choroid is also thin throughout.

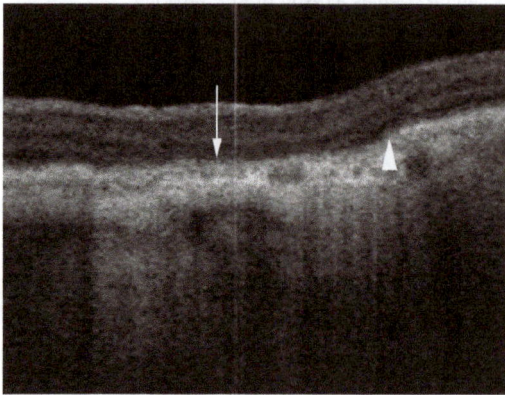

Fig. 5.7. Magnified view of the white box in Fig. 5.4. Attenuation of the RPE line (*arrowhead*) with thinning of the inner retina and disruption of normal outer retina anatomy is seen (*arrow*). Thin choroid is a characteristic finding in patients with AMD.

Neovascular Age-related Macular Degeneration

Neovascular AMD is characterized by choroidal neovascularization (CNV) which may occur above or below the RPE. Common accompanying features include pigment epithelial detachments (PED), intraretinal and subretinal fluid (SRF).

Classic Choroidal Neovascularization

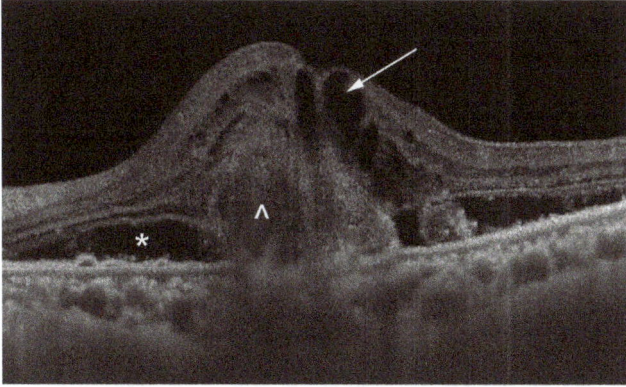

Fig. 5.8. SSOCT scan (cut represented by long white arrow across Fig. 5.9) of a patient with type II CNV which shows the presence of SRF (*white asterisk*) and macula cyst (*arrow*). A subfoveal hyperreflective lesion localized within the subretinal space (^) above the RPE, representing a type II CNV, is seen on SS-OCT. This corresponds to the area of classic leakage pattern on FFA (Fig. 5.10).

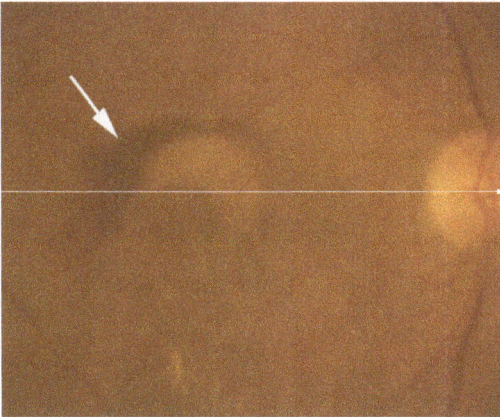

Fig. 5.9. Corresponding color photo to Fig. 5.8, showing subretinal blood (*white arrow*).

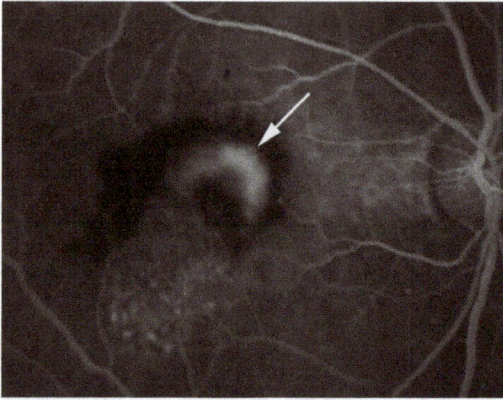

Fig. 5.10. Corresponding FFA to Fig. 5.8, showing early phase hyperflourescent lesion (*white arrow*).

Occult Choroidal Neovascularization

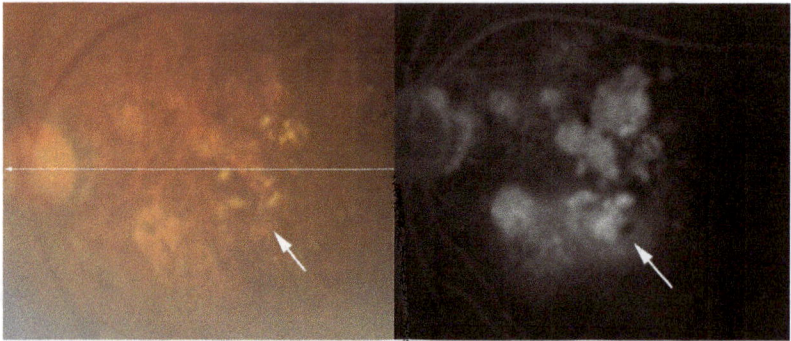

Fig. 5.11. Color fundus photo (on the *left*) showing drusen and patchy areas of hypopigmentation (*white arrow*) and FFA (on the *right*) showing late leakage from a fibrovascular PED (*white arrow*).

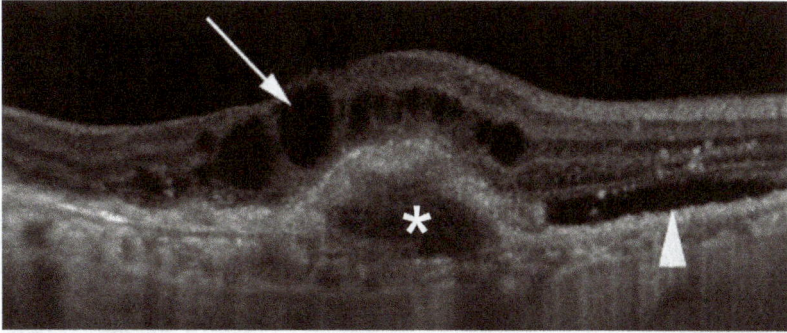

Fig. 5.12. SS-OCT scan (cut represented by long white arrow across Fig. 5.11) shows clear delineation of the RPE layer despite hazy media and asteroid hyalosis in this patient. The sub RPE hyper-reflective lesion (*asterisk*) and the presence of hyperreflective material on the undersurface of PED suggest a fibrovascular PED. Overlying retinal cysts (*arrow*) and adjacent subretinal fluid (*arrowhead*) are seen. FFA (Fig. 5.11) shows a corresponding area of late leakage, confirming the diagnosis of occult CNV.

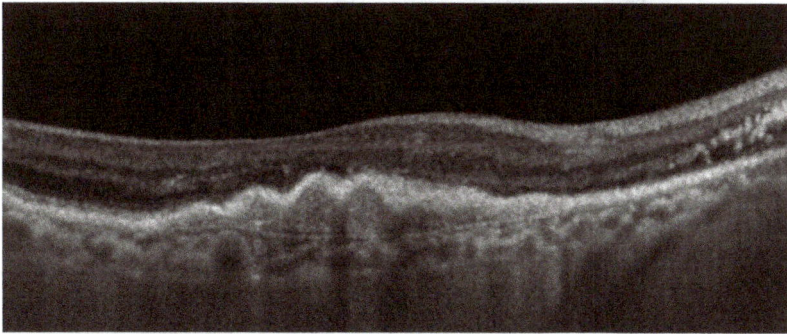

Fig. 5.13. One month after treatment with intravitreal anti-VEGF, both intraretinal and subretinal fluid have resolved.

Polypoidal Choroidal Vasculopathy

Polypoidal choroidal vasculopathy (PCV) is a disorder involving the inner choroidal circulation characterized by the presence of polypoidal, subretinal branching vascular network with aneurysmal terminals. Clinically, it appears as polyp-like orange nodules. It often presents as multiple, recurrent serosanguineous retinal pigment epithelial and neurosensory detachment (Fig. 5.14) due to the leakage or bleeding from the lesions.

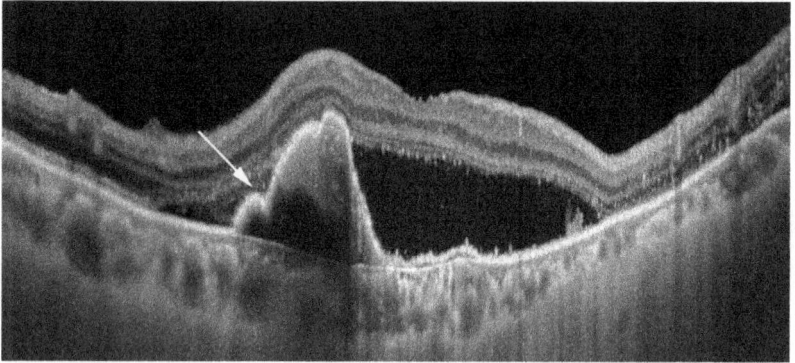

Fig. 5.14. SS-OCT scan (cut represented by long white arrow across Fig. 5.16) shows the presence of "double humps sign" (*white arrow*) associated with subretinal fluid.

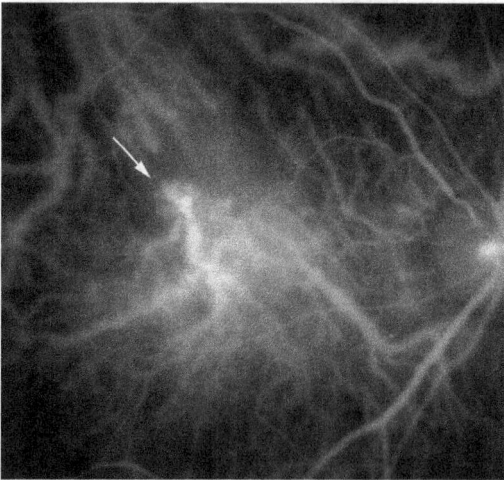

Fig. 5.15. Indocyanine green angiogram (ICGA), presence of hyperflourescent nodules (*white arrow*) which persisted into the late phase.

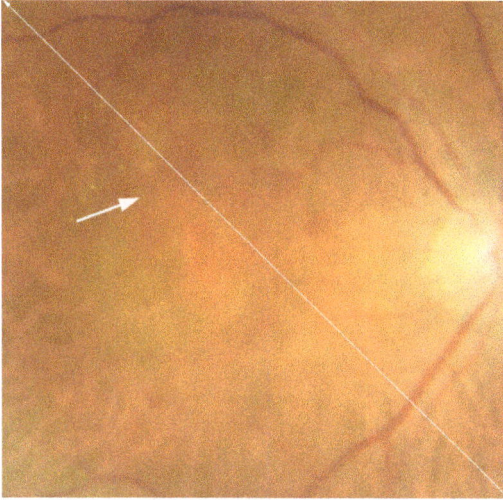

Fig. 5.16. Presence of orange-red nodule (*white arrow*) in color fundus photos.

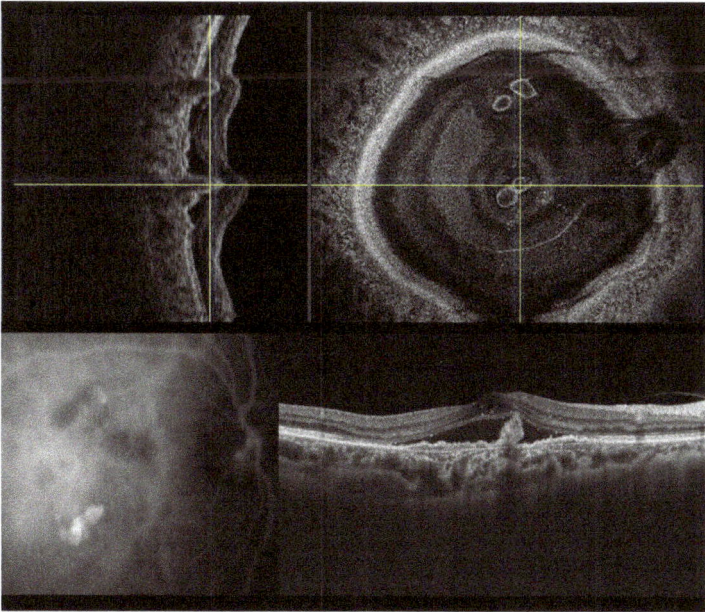

Fig. 5.17. Top images show the enface scan of a PCV with subretinal fluid with corresponding ICG angiogram showing PCV as hotspots (*bottom left*) and longitudinal scan (*bottom right*) with SS-OCT.

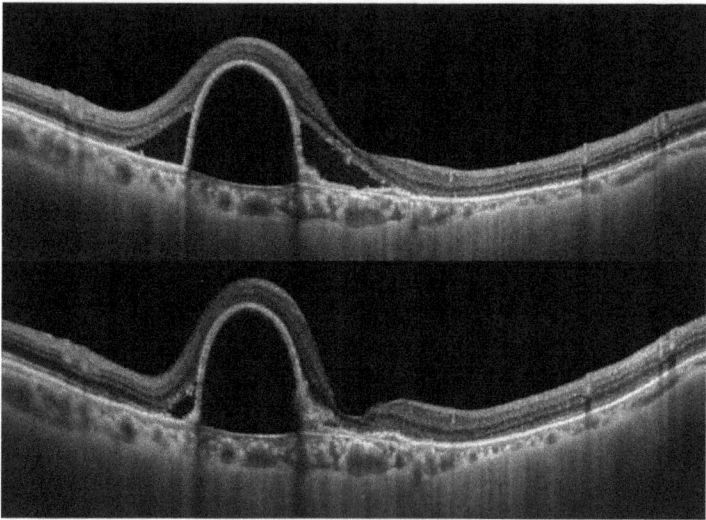

Fig. 5.18. Shows treatment of PCV with combination therapy of photodynamic therapy and anti-vascular endothelial growth factor (anti-VEGF). Top image shows 3 months post-treatment and bottom image shows 6 months post-treatment. Notice the reduction in subretinal fluid; however, the PED is still persistent.

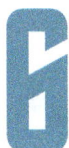

6 VITREO MACULAR INTERFACE DISEASE

Epiretinal Membrane

Epiretinal membrane (ERM) is cellular proliferation on the inner retinal surface (Fig. 6.1). The symptoms of ERM may range from asymptomatic to debilitating metamorphopsia and central visual loss. The etiology is often idiopathic in nature while some secondary causes include retinal tear/retinal detachment, retinal vascular diseases, inflammation, trauma, previous retinal lasers and retinitis pigmentosa.

Grading of ERM

Grade 0 (cellophane maculopathy): a translucent membrane with no underlying retinal distortion

Grade 1 (wrinkled cellophane maculopathy): ERM with irregular wrinkling of the inner retina

Grade 2 (macular pucker): an opaque membrane causing obscuration of underlying vessels and marked full-thickness retinal distortion.

Treatment

Conservative — benign, asymptomatic patients

Surgery — pars plana vitrectomy, epiretinal membrane and inner limiting membrane peeling with/or without membrane staining.

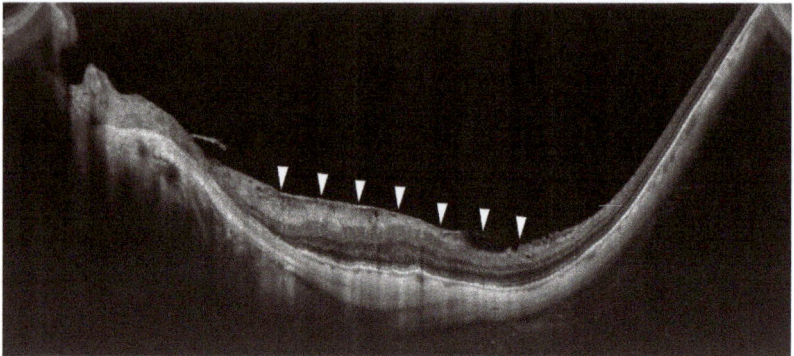

Fig. 6.1. SS-OCT shows epiretinal membrane (*white arrows*) in a high myope patient with posterior staphyloma.

Macular Hole

A macular hole (MH) is a retinal break involving the fovea. It is usually idiopathic but may be associated with myopia, epiretinal membrane and trauma. Suggested pathophysiology includes tangential traction and anterior-posterior traction of the posterior hyaloid on the parafovea. Up to 30% of patients have bilateral macular holes. The most common symptoms are metamorphopsia and central scotoma, and a positive Watzke-Allen's test (perception of a "break" in the middle of the slit beam) is helpful in making the diagnosis.

Macula holes can be divided into 4 stages

Stage 1a: Foveal detachment (yellow dot stage)

Stage 1b: Yellow ring

Stage 2: Full thickness macula hole (<400 µm)

Stage 3: Full thickness macula hole (>400 µm) with partial vitreomacular traction (VMT)

Stage 4: Full thickness macula hole (>400 µm) with posterior vitreous detachment.

Treatment

Conservative

Surgical — can be considered for stage 2 or higher:

Pars plana vitrectomy with epiretinal and inner limiting membrane peeling and endotamponade with/or without triamcinolone and membrane staining.

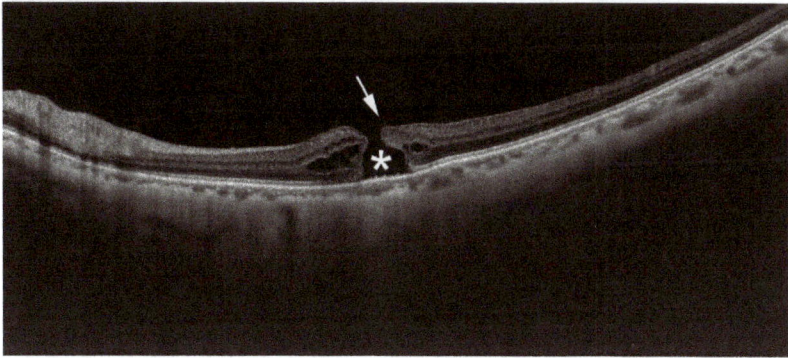

Fig. 6.2. SS-OCT shows presence of a full thickness macula hole (*) with vitreomacular traction (*white arrow*).

Vitreomacular Traction

Vitreomacular traction (VMT) (Fig. 6.3) is a vitreoretinal interface disorder characterized by an incomplete posterior vitreous detachment, with the persistently adherent vitreous over the macula, resulting in morphologic alterations and consequent decline of visual function. With age, there is a sequential weakening of attachments between the vitreous and the internal limiting membrane (starting from the perifoveal region), superior and inferior vascular arcades, fovea, mid-peripheral retina then optic disc.

Based on the diameter of vitreous attachment to the macular surface measured by OCT, the International Vitrecomacular Traction Study Group sub-classified VMT into focal (1500 μm or less) or broad (1500 μm or more).

Treatment

Conservative — asymptomatic or mildly symptomatic patient with good visual acuity

Surgery — pars plana vitrectomy combined with ERM peeling with/ or without ILM peeling and gas endotamponade

New agents — ocriplasmin.

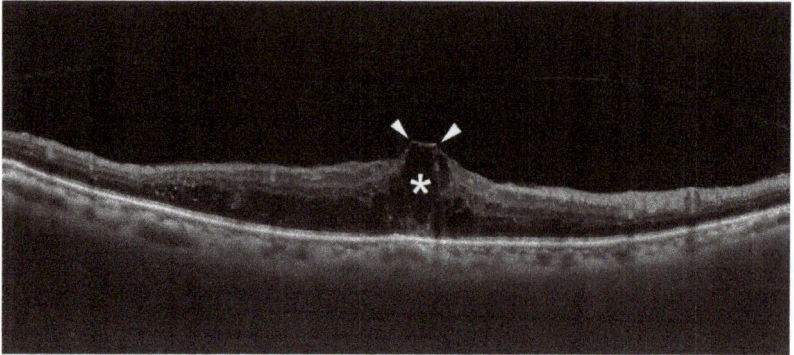

Fig. 6.3. SS-OCT shows vitreomacular traction (VMT) denoted by 2 white arrows and cystoid macular edema (*).

7 MYOPIA

Pathologic Myopia

Pathologic myopia is defined as high myopia accompanied by characteristic degenerative changes in the sclera, choroid, RPE and compromised visual function mostly in those with -6 dioptres or worse and axial length of 26.0 mm or longer.

Common degenerative changes include a tessellated fundus, chorioretinal atrophy (Fig. 7.2), lacquer cracks (Fig. 7.3), and posterior staphyloma. Factors such as vitreal-macula traction (Fig. 7.5), posterior staphyloma and scleral stretching are thought to contribute to posterior pole abnormalities such as myopic foveoschisis (Fig. 7.5), fovea detachment (Fig. 7.6) choroidal neovascularization (Fig. 7.7), and dome-shaped macula (Fig. 7.4).

SS-OCT provides an accurate high definition transverse image of these retinal changes, allowing for prompt diagnosis and severity of the condition. Compared with SDOCT, SS-OCT has greater sensitivity and lower signal-to-noise ratio (SNR) at greater scanning depths. In addition, the enface scan function of the SS-OCT can help localize and determine the lateral extent of these changes.

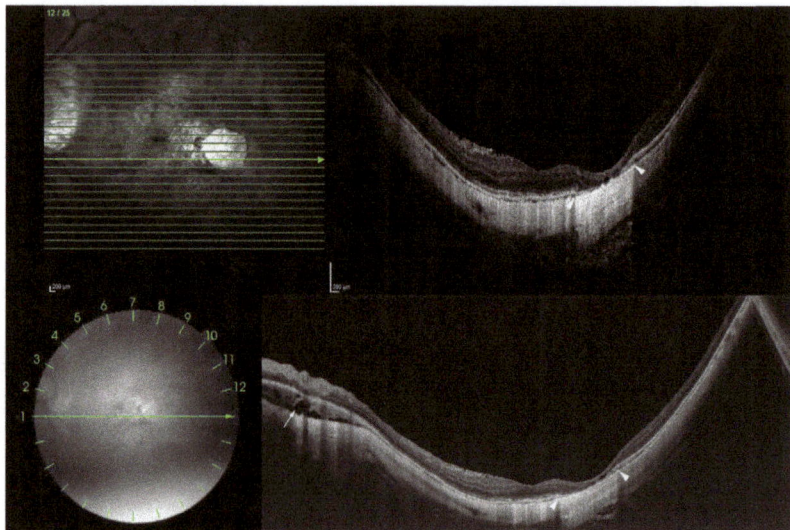

Fig. 7.1. SS-OCT *vs.* SD-OCT. Closest corresponding scans between SS-OCT and SDOCT are compared here. The useable area of the SS-OCT scan is 10.9 mm (*bottom*) as compared to the area imaged by SD-OCT at 8 mm. In addition, the SS-OCT scan has greater sensitivity and lower signal-to-noise ratio (SNR) than the SD-OCT. Although a wider area is imaged in SS-OCT scans, mirror artifacts are seen. Features seen here on both scans include an area of retinal atrophy and increased signal transmission (*between arrowheads*); however, intrachoroidal cavitation is much better appreciated on SS-OCT (arrow) but can barely be seen on SD-OCT.

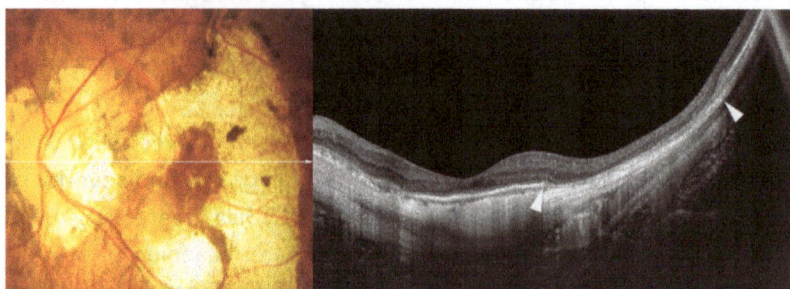

Fig. 7.2. Chorioretinal atrophy. Area of chorioretinal atrophy as seen in color fundus photography with corresponding SS-OCT scan (*area between the 2 white arrows*). SS-OCT *scan* (cut represented by long white arrow across color fundal photo) shows a thin choroid and decreased retinal thickness. This is in contrast to areas of normal retina beyond the 2 white arrows.

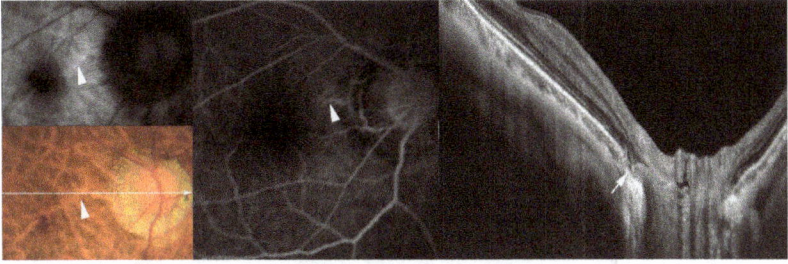

Fig. 7.3. Lacquer crack. Top *left* images shows autofluorescence (AF) image and color fundus photo of lacquer crack (*white arrows*) just temporal to the optic disc. Middle image shows late hyperfluorescence staining of lacquer crack on fluorescein angiogram. Corresponding SS-OCT scan (cut represented by long white arrow across color fundal photo) shows disruption in the retinal pigment epithelium (*right image, white arrow*).

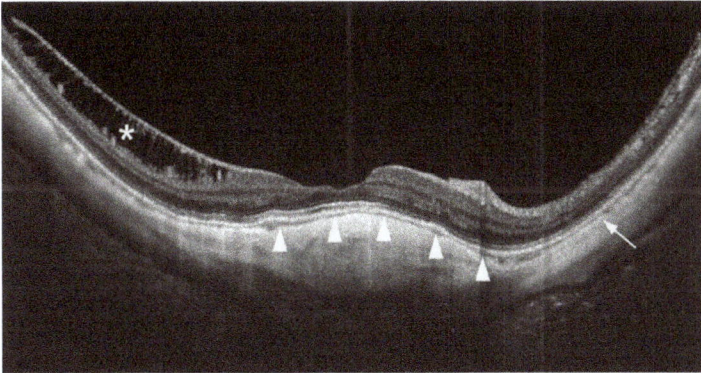

Fig. 7.4. Dome-shaped macula. Longitudinal SS-OCT image of myopic fundus. The SS-OCT scan is still able to image the posterior limit of a myopic fundus, including the sclera and choroid with good resolution. The domed-shaped macula is denoted by the white arrows. There is an area of retinoschisis (*). Note also the thin choroid (*arrow*).

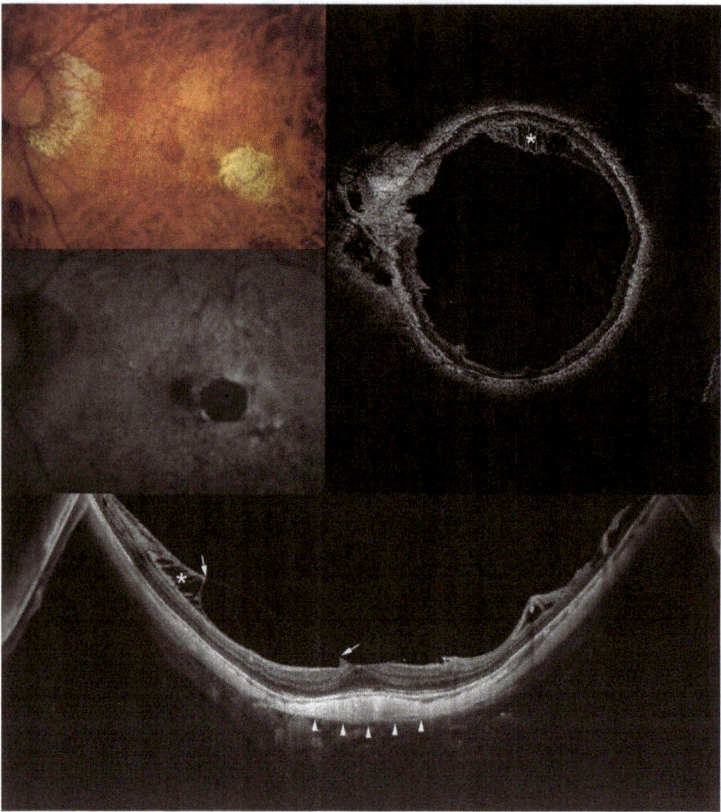

Fig. 7.5. Vitreomacular traction, retinoschisis. Top *left* images shows color fundus photo and AF images of eye with multiple myopic pathology. On SS-OCT longitudinal scan (*bottom*), VMT is clearly visualized (*white arrows with tails*), resulting in retinoschisis (denoted by *), showing strands of intraretinal bridges. Enface scan (*top right*) shows the intraretinal schisis as a honeycomb pattern (denoted by *).

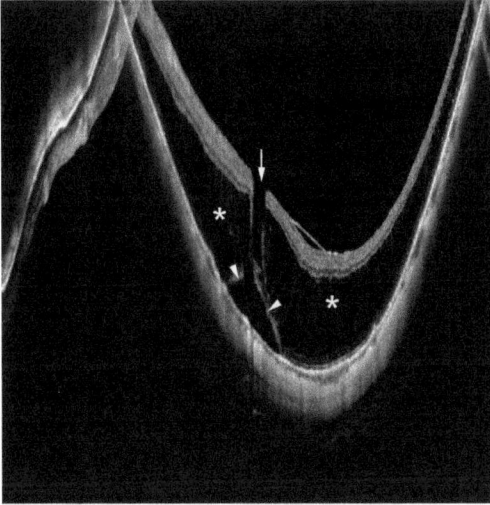

Fig. 7.6. Foveoschisis with fovea detachment and macula hole. This longitudinal SS-OCT scan shows foveoschisis (*) with fovea detachment (*white arrowheads*) and a macula hole (*white arrow*).

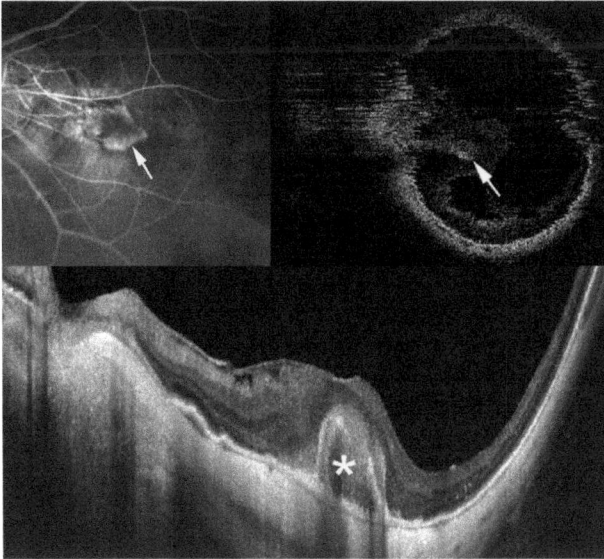

Fig. 7.7. Myopic CNV. Top *left* image shows FFA of myopic CNV lesion (*white arrows*). This corresponds to the enface image on SS-OCT (*top right*) and longitudinal OCT scan (*bottom*). CNV lesion is denoted by (*).

8 INFLAMMATORY CONDITIONS

Vogt-Koyanagi-Harada (VKH) Syndrome

VKH is a multisystem disorder characterized by granulomatous uveitis, often associated with neurologic and cutaneous manifestations. Ocular features include exudative retinal detachments in the acute phase and "sunset-glow" appearance in the chronic phase, resulting from depigmentation.

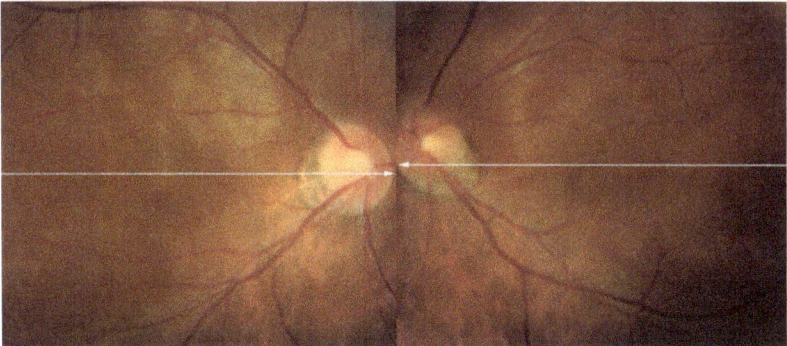

Fig. 8.1. Color fundus photo showing acute VKH with multifocal serous retinal detachments.

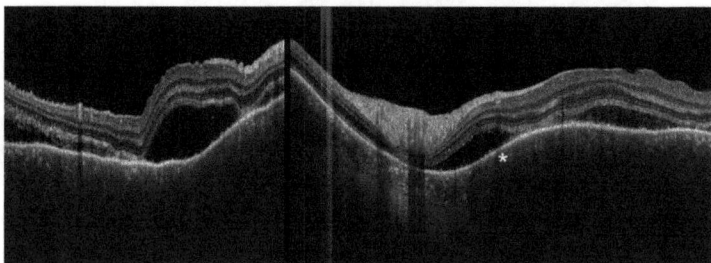

Fig. 8.2. SSOCT *scan* (cut represented by long white arrow across Fig. 8.1) shows presence of serous retinal detachments and RPE undulations due to underlying choroidal inflammation, as well as thickened choroid suggestive of choroidal inflammation. In these scans, the choroid is so thickened (*), the choroid-sclera interface cannot be seen.

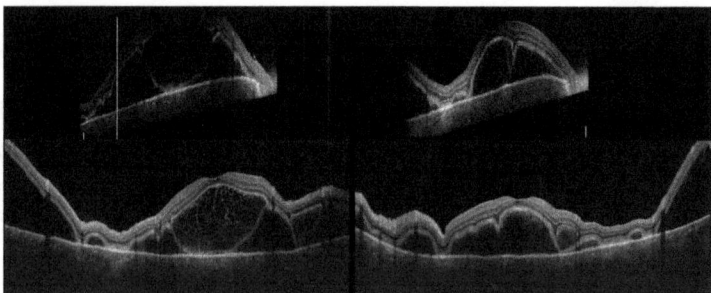

Fig. 8.3. This case demonstrates the differences between SS-OCT (*bottom row*) and SDOCT (*top row*). In the SS-OCT scans (*bottom row*) the extent and depth of detachments are better appreciated from the longer and deeper scans achieved with SS-OCT. In addition, subretinal fibrinous material and septae are also better appreciated on the higher resolution SS-OCT scans. Choroidal thickness, however, cannot be assessed even with SS-OCT at baseline.

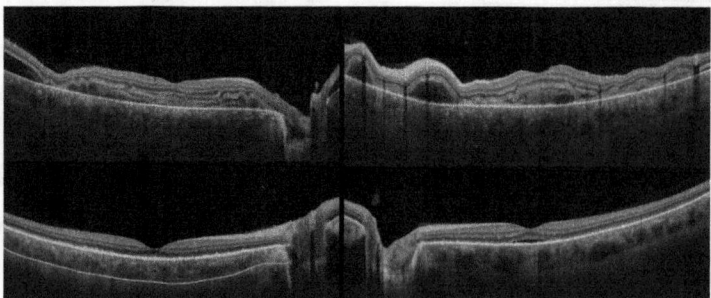

Fig. 8.4. These SS-OCT scans demonstrate the resolution of neurosensory detachment and normalization of thickened choroid. *Top* row scans show results of treatment after 3 days of intravenous methylprednisolone, and *bottom* row scans show results after 1 month.

Chorioretinitis

Chorioretinitis (CR) is an inflammatory process of the uveal tract of the eye and can be caused by inflammatory or infective etiologies such as bacterial, viral or fungal. Congenital toxoplasma is a common etiology in the neonatal age group.

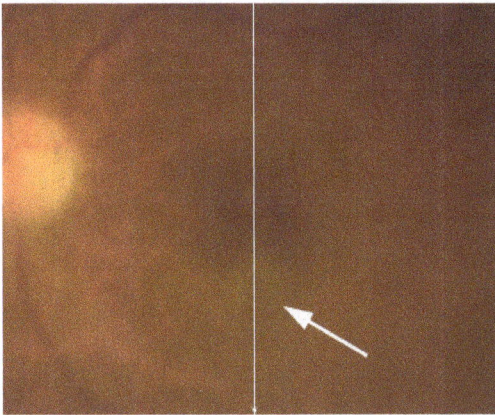

Fig. 8.5. Color fundus photo of toxoplasmosis chorioretinitis. Shows a greyish white raised lesion inferior to the fovea (*white arrow*).

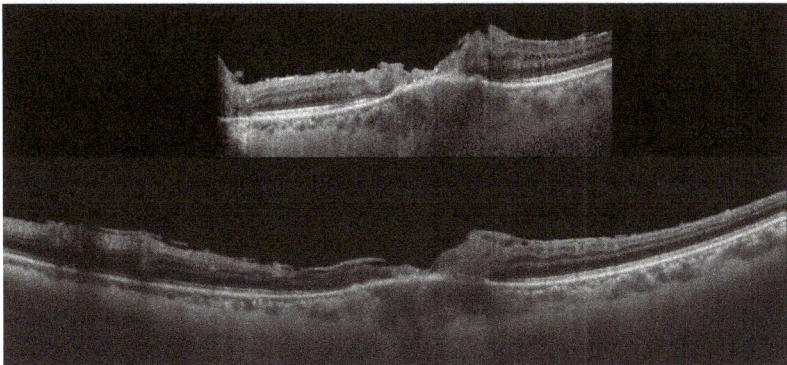

Fig. 8.6. Toxoplasmosis chorioretinitis. Comparison between SDOCT scan (*top*) and SS-OCT scan (*bottom*) shows the larger extent, depth and resolution, SS-OCT has over SDOCT. In both scans, the area of retinitis is imaged as a raised disorganized lesion, with loss of normal retina architecture. There is a thinning of the retina, loss of normal striations, and a disorganized RPE.

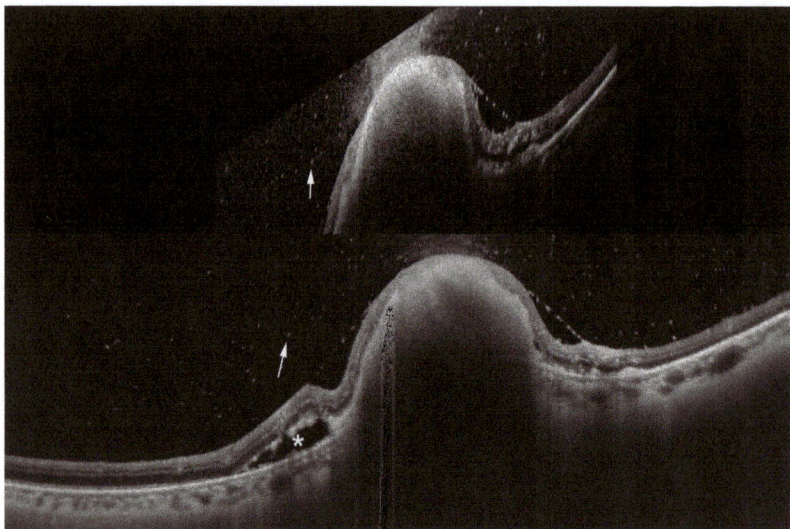

Fig. 8.7. Fungal chorioretinal abscess. Another comparison is demonstrated here between SDOCT scan (*top*) and SS-OCT scan (*bottom*) of a fungal chorioretinal abscess. In addition to the domed-shaped abscess evident on both scans, the larger extent and depth of the SS-OCT scan shows the presence of a neurosensory detachment adjacent to the lesion (*) that is not seen on the SDOCT. In both scans, there is presence of vitritis seen as hyperreflective spots in the vitreous (*white arrow*).

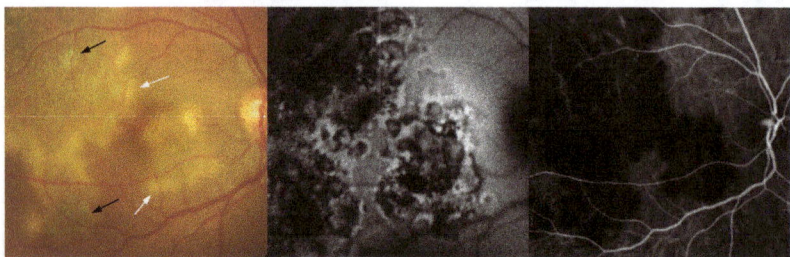

Fig. 8.8. Tubercular serpiginous-like choroiditis. Color fundus photo (*left*) showing foveal-equatorial yellow white patchy lesion (*white arrows*), with peripheral edges showing hyperpigmentation (*black arrows*) which spar the disc. The extent of the lesion is better defined on autofluorescence (*middle*). ICGA (*right*) shows greater sensitivity in defining the extent of subclinical lesions. Areas of hypofluorescence on ICGA could represent blocked fluorescence from diseased RPE.

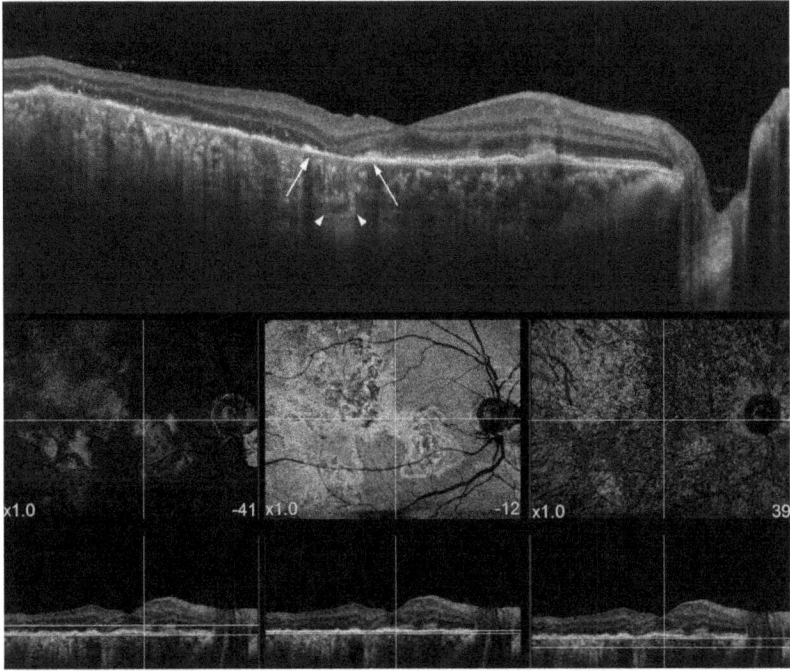

Fig. 8.9. Tuberculosis-associated pigment epitheliopathy. SSOCT *scan* (top; cut represented by long white arrow across Fig. 8.8) shows relatively well preserved RPE, with disruption of the outer retinal layers and EZ. Other areas showing increased reflectance throughout the outer nuclear layer (*between white arrowheads*) correspond to the white lesions on fundal color photos, AF and ICGA. The edge of these lesions have areas of pigment clumping (*white arrows*).

Enface view of the outer retina (*bottom left*) shows areas of hyperreflectivity as in the enface view of the RPE level (*bottom middle*), where hyperreflective areas surrounding hyporeflective spots represent irregular thickening of the RPE. Enface view of the choroid (*bottom right*) shows areas of hyperreflectivity corresponding to areas of increased transmission possibly through deficient RPE and outer retinal layers.

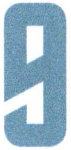

9 MISCELLANEOUS CONDITIONS

Choroidal Hemangioma

The choroidal hemangioma is a benign vascular tumor of the choroid. The circumscribed form is isolated and non-syndromic, while the diffuse form is usually part of the Sturge–Weber syndrome. Visual symptoms are caused by exudative retinal detachment or degenerative changes in the macula. Treatment options include photodynamic therapy, transpupillary thermotherapy, radiation therapy or enucleation for painful blind eyes.

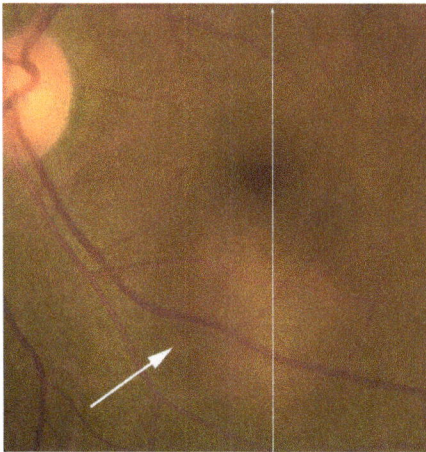

Fig. 9.1. A pale subretinal lesion which represents a circumscribed choroidal hemangioma is seen along the inferotemporal quadrant.

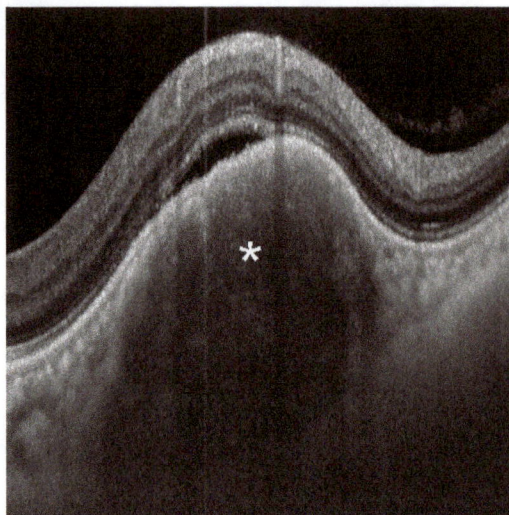

Fig. 9.2. SS-OCT (cut represented by long white arrow across Fig. 9.1) shows a smooth, dome-shaped elevation of the choroidal tumor. There is also acoustic shadowing and expansion of the choriocapillary network. An overlying pocket of subretinal fluid is seen.

Choroidal Naevus

Choroidal nevi are the most common intraocular tumor seen in ophthalmic practice. It is a benign melanocytic tumor that is commonly seen after puberty. Choroidal nevi is often asymptomatic and seen posterior to the equator. The clinical appearance is a brown or slate grey lesion that is flat or minimally elevated. It is occasionally associated with drusen or serous detachment of the sensory retina.

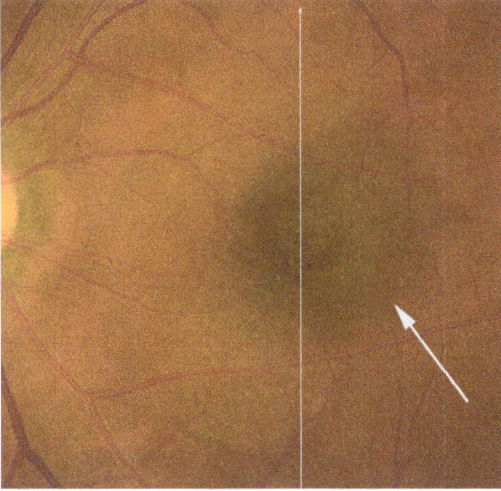

Fig. 9.3. Color fundus photo showing the choroidal nevus involving the macula (*white arrow*).

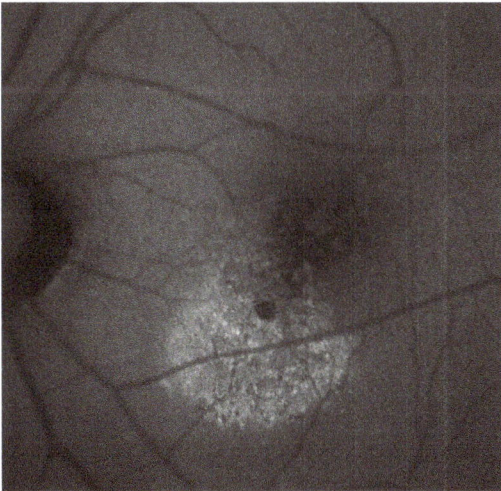

Fig. 9.4. Fundus autofluorescence showing hyperflourescent areas suggestive of retinal pigment epithelium dysfunction.

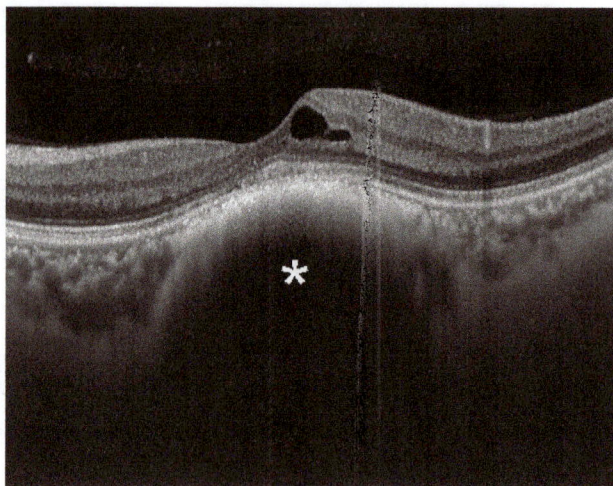

Fig. 9.5. SS-OCT scan (cut represented by long white arrow across Fig. 9.3) showing subfoveal choroidal nevus and overlying intraretinal cystoid changes. This image clearly shows the vitreous anatomy.

Focal Choroidal Excavation (FCE)

FCE is a newly described clinical idiopathic entity, which manifests as thinning of the choroid. Vision is usually minimally affected. However, it can be associated with central serous chorioretinopathy, choroidal neovascularization, epiretinal membrane and age-related macular degeneration. OCT is the optimal imaging modality for diagnosis.

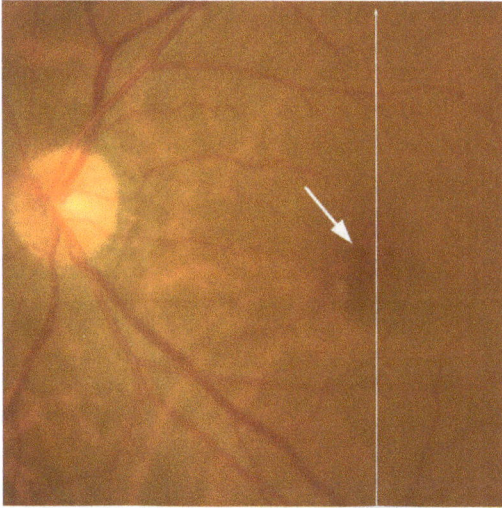

Fig. 9.6. Left eye showing mottling at the macula and retinal pigment epithelium disturbance (*white arrow*).

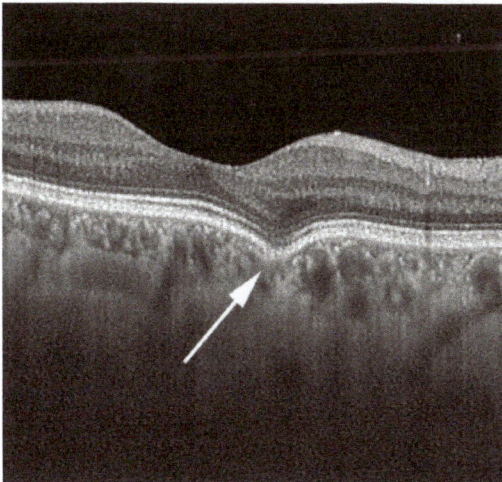

Fig. 9.7. SS-OCT scan (cut represented by long white arrow across Fig. 9.6) of the left posterior pole, showing thinned out choroidal tissue just beneath the area of FCE (*arrow*). This thinned out choroidal tissue has high internal reflectivity and there is poor visualization of both the medium and large diameter choroidal vessels. There is loss of contour of the outer choroidal boundary, which appears to be pulled inwards by this abnormal choroidal tissue.

Optic Pit with Neurosensory Detachment

Optic pits are congenital excavations of the optic nerve head with no gender predilection, and are usually sporadic. They are often asymptomatic unless complicated by macular edema, schisis or serous detachment.

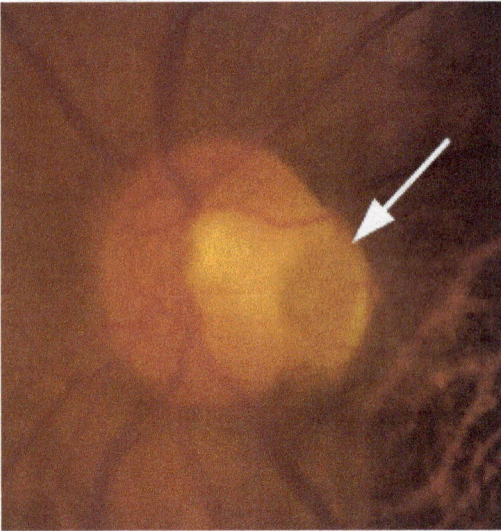

Fig. 9.8. Optic pit. This optic pit appears as a small oval excavated depression in the optic nerve head. Optic pits are most commonly located on the temporal side of the optic disc (as in this case), but they may be situated anywhere along the margin of the optic disc.

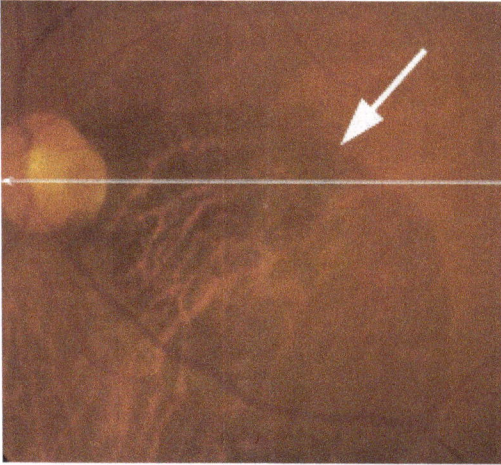

Fig. 9.9. Optic pit with serous detachment. This optic pit, which is along the rim of the optic disc, has led to serous detachment of the retina involving the macula (*white arrow*).

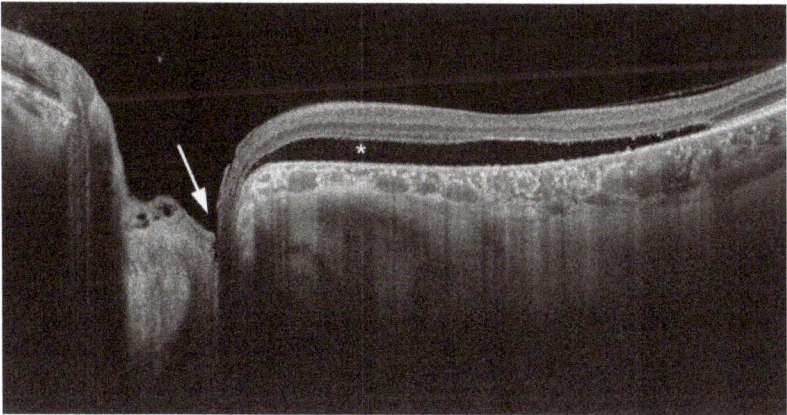

Fig. 9.10. SSOCT scan of optic pit with serous detachment. This SSOCT scan (cut represented by long white arrow across Fig. 9.9) shows the extent of serous detachment (*) originating from the optic pit (*white arrow*).

Morning Glory Disc

It is a congenital, funnel-shaped excavation of the posterior fundus that incorporates the optic disc. The disc is enlarged with a central glial tuft. The surrounding retinal vessels are anomalous and there is surrounding peripapillary chorioretinal pigmentary disturbance. It is often unilateral with a female preponderance. Ocular complications include serous or rhegmatogenous retinal detachment, or choroidal neovascularization. Systemic associations include trans-sphenoidal basal encephalocele, corpus callosum agenesis and septo-optic dysplasia.

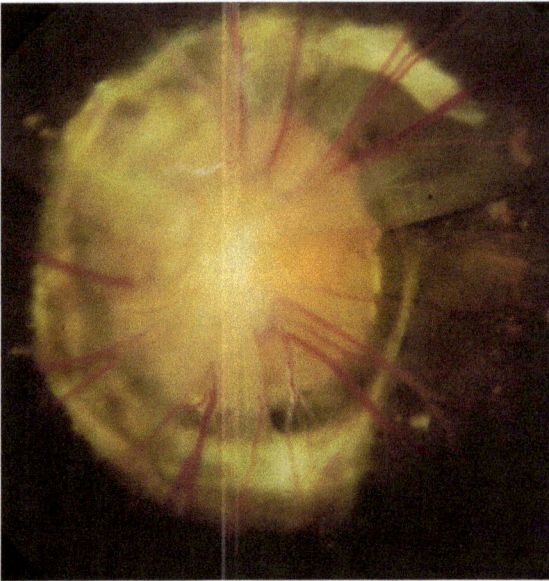

Fig. 9.11. Morning glory disc showing enlarged and excavated optic disc. The surrounding retinal vessels are in a spoke-like arrangement and there is an overlying tuft of glial tissue.

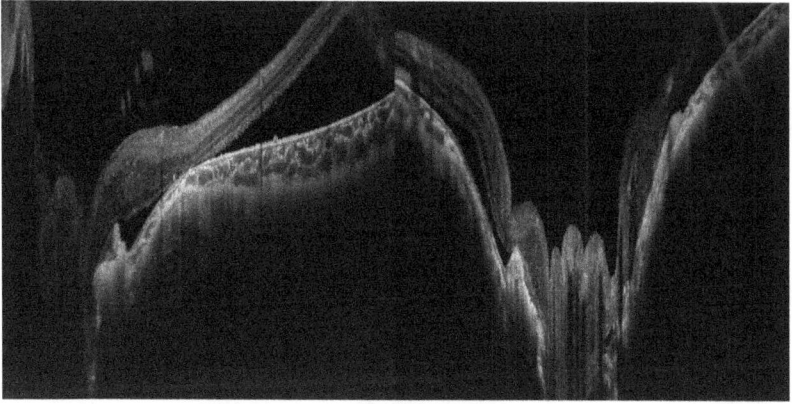

Fig. 9.12. SS-OCT showing an excavated optic disc with surrounding retinal detachment.

INDEX